RELIEVING TIGHT HIP FLEXORS

A Comprehensive Guide to Practical Exercises, Stretching Routines, and Lifestyle Adjustments for Optimal Hip Health and Pain-Free Movement

By

Sharon G. Brown

TABLE OF CONTENT

INTRODUCTION

Are you frustrated with the challenges and physical restrictions that come with having tight hip flexors? Are you struggling to maintain an active and pain-free lifestyle? "Relieving Tight Hip Flexors" is filled with detailed explanations, vibrant illustrations, and practical advice, all aimed at giving you the tools to manage your hip health. If you're seeking to enhance your athletic performance, relieve discomfort, or simply move more effortlessly, this guide will equip you with the necessary resources. By utilizing the information provided, you can restore your flexibility, enhance your strength, and experience a rejuvenated outlook on life.

This guide provides a thorough and captivating exploration of the hip flexors, shedding light on their significance in various aspects of your body, such as posture and athletic abilities. Whether you're an athlete, a desk worker, or simply someone seeking relief from chronic discomfort, this book provides valuable insights and practical solutions.

What does it contain?

- Anatomy of the Hip Flexors: A comprehensive understanding of the role that hip flexors play in your body. The inner workings of these systems, the factors that contribute to their tightness, and the effects this can have on your overall well-being and range of motion.

- Identifying Tight Hip Flexors: Uncertain about the source of your hip flexor issues? We'll provide you with step-by-step instructions on how to effectively assess your body for tightness and imbalances.

- Stretching and Strengthening Routines: Bid farewell to one-size-fits-all recommendations. Explore a range of exercises and routines that have been carefully crafted to effectively alleviate tension and enhance the strength of your hip flexors. These straightforward plans will assist you in attaining enduring flexibility and resilience.

- Effective techniques for performing Myofascial Release at home using foam rollers and other tools. Thorough, systematic instructions that will help you effectively alleviate muscle tightness and enhance blood circulation.

- A range of Yoga Poses and Pilates Exercises designed to enhance hip flexibility and strengthen your core. Incorporate these practices into your daily routine to experience comprehensive health benefits.

- The impact of making minor adjustments to your daily routine on maintaining hip health and preventing future issues. From ergonomic tips to adopting an active lifestyle, discover the power of small changes for long-term relief.

This guide goes beyond a mere compilation of exercises, it provides a thorough guide to regaining your ability to move freely. Eliminate the limitations caused by tight hip flexors and enhance your health and well-being by investing in " Relieving Tight Hip Flexors" and embark on a path towards increased flexibility, strength, and vitality.

CHAPTER ONE

Anatomy of the Hip Flexors

The hip flexors are a group of muscles that have a significant impact on the movement and stability of the hip joint. These muscles play a crucial role in the movement of the hip, specifically in bringing the thigh closer to the torso. Gaining a thorough understanding of the hip flexors' anatomy is crucial in identifying any problems associated with tightness, pain, and limitations in mobility. Presented is a thorough examination of the primary muscles that make up the hip flexors and their respective roles.

The Major Hip Flexor Muscles

1. The Iliopsoas Muscle Group

Here are some anatomical terms related to the muscles in the hip and thigh:

- Iliacus

- Psoas Major

- Psoas Minor

2. Rectus Femoris
3. Sartorius
4. The Tensor Fasciae Latae (TFL) muscle
5. The pectineus muscle is a small but important muscle located in the hip region.
6. The adductor group

1. The Iliopsoas Muscle Group

The Iliacus muscles

The iliacus muscle is derived from the iliac fossa, which is located on the inner surface of the ilium, a large pelvic bone. It is located in the lesser trochanter of the femur. The iliacus muscle is responsible for flexing and externally rotating the thigh. It engages in various movements like walking, running, and bending at the hip.

The Psoas Major

The psoas major muscle originates from the transverse processes, bodies, and intervertebral discs of the T12 to L5 vertebrae. Additionally, it connects to the lesser trochanter of the femur, linking the iliacus.

This muscle is responsible for flexing the hip joint and providing stability to the spine and pelvis. Understanding the importance of activities such as lifting the leg and maintaining posture is essential.

The Psoas Minor

The psoas minor is a smaller muscle that originates from the bodies of T12 and L1 vertebrae. It is sometimes absent and is located in the iliopubic eminence.

The psoas minor plays a role in flexing the lumbar spine, although it is not the main muscle responsible for hip flexion.

2. Rectus Femoris

The rectus femoris is located within the quadriceps femoris group and it originates from the anterior inferior iliac spine and the groove above the acetabulum. The insertion point is located in the patellar tendon, which is connected to the tibial tuberosity.

The rectus femoris is responsible for flexing the hip and extending the knee. The quadriceps muscle is crucial for performing actions such as kicking and jumping, as it crosses both the hip and knee joints.

3. Sartorius

The sartorius muscle holds the distinction of being the longest muscle in the human body. It comes from the anterior superior iliac spine. The insertion point is located on the medial aspect of the proximal tibia, which is part of the pes anserinus group.

The sartorius muscle performs several functions, including hip flexion, abduction, and external rotation, as well as knee flexion. This muscle is responsible for various activities, including crossing the legs and running.

4. Tensor Fasciae Latae (TFL)

The TFL is located at the origin point of the anterior iliac crest and the anterior superior iliac spine. The insertion point is located in the iliotibial (IT) band, which extends along the outer side of the thigh to the lateral tibial condyle.

The TFL contributes to hip flexion, abduction, and internal rotation. Additionally, it aids in maintaining stability in the pelvis and knee while engaging in activities such as walking and running.

5. Pectineus

The pectineus muscle is situated at the pectineal line of the pubis. It is located at the pectineal line of the femur. The pectineus muscle is responsible for flexing and adducting the hip. It plays a crucial role in facilitating movements that bring the thighs closer and providing stability to the hip joint.

6. The Adductor Group

It consists of the adductor brevis, adductor longus, and adductor magnus muscles. These muscles have their origins at different points on the pubis and ischium. They are inserted along the linea aspera of the femur.

The adductor muscles play a crucial role in hip adduction and also assist in hip flexion, particularly when the hip is already flexed.

The Function and Importance of The Hip Flexors

The involvement of the hip flexors in numerous daily activities and sports is significant. They have a crucial function in:

- Walking and running: Examining the flexion of the hip to elevate the leg.

- Sitting and standing: Bringing the thigh closer to the torso.

- Physical Activities: Engaging in movements such as kicking, jumping, and making rapid changes in direction.

Common Problems with Hip Flexors

- Tightness and shortening: Extended periods of sitting or neglecting to stretch can result in tight hip flexors, which can cause discomfort and limit your range of motion.

- Strains and injuries can be quite common and can occur due to various reasons. Excessive or abrupt movements can cause strain on the hip flexors, resulting in discomfort and reduced strength.

- Tight hip flexors can have a significant impact on posture, leading to an anterior pelvic tilt and causing lower back pain. This can greatly affect overall posture and biomechanics.

Gaining a deep understanding of the hip flexors' anatomy offers valuable insights into their pivotal role in both movement and stability. By implementing a routine of stretching, strengthening, and mindful movement, one can effectively preserve the functionality of their body and minimize the risk of tightness and injury. Having a solid understanding of this fundamental knowledge is crucial for individuals seeking to enhance their hip health and overall mobility.

Possible Factors Contributing to Tight Hip Flexors

Many individuals, regardless of age or activity level, often experience the problem of tight hip flexors. Gaining a thorough understanding of the causes can be instrumental in preventing and effectively addressing the problem. These are a few of the most prevalent causes:

> **Sitting for extended periods of time:**

Extended periods of sitting, whether at a desk, in a car, or on the couch, can lead to the shortening and tightening of the hip flexors. The reason for this is that the hip flexors stay in a shortened position when you sit.

Work environment: Occupations that involve prolonged periods of sitting without regular breaks may contribute to the development of persistent muscle tightness.

> ### **Insufficient or lack of Stretching:**

Overlooking Flexibility Training: Numerous individuals prioritize strength training while disregarding stretching, resulting in muscle imbalances and tight hip flexors.

Insufficient Stretching: Even individuals who engage in regular exercise may not prioritize stretching enough to adequately maintain flexibility in the hip flexors.

> ### **Repetitive Movements:**

Engaging in sports and activities that require frequent hip flexion, like running, cycling, and specific gym exercises, can put excessive strain on the hip flexors.

Occupational Hazards: Certain jobs that require repetitive motions, such as bending and lifting, can contribute to muscle tightness.

> **Posture Issues:**

When sitting with a rounded back and poor posture, there is an increased strain on the hip flexors.

Posture: When standing, it's important to be mindful of the position of your pelvis. Tilting it forward can lead to tightness in the hip flexors.

> **Muscle Imbalances:**

When the muscles on the back of the hip are weak, it can lead to overactivity and tightness in the hip flexors as a compensatory mechanism.

One potential issue to be aware of is a weak core, which can result in suboptimal pelvic alignment and a greater dependence on the hip flexors for stability.

> **Injury or Overuse**

When the hip flexors or surrounding muscles are injured, the body may tighten up as a protective measure.

Excessive training or inadequate rest can lead to overuse injuries, resulting in tightness in the hip flexors.

Symptoms and Impact on Daily Life

Having tight hip flexors can cause a variety of symptoms and have a significant impact on your daily activities. Presented below are several typical symptoms and their corresponding impacts:

> **Pain and Discomfort:**

Tight hip flexors can contribute to or worsen lower back pain by pulling the pelvis forward, which puts additional strain on the lumbar spine.

Pain in the hip area, particularly when there is movement or stretching of the hip flexors.

Thigh Pain: Pain may be experienced in the front of the thigh as a result of tight hip flexors.

> **Limitations in Movement:**

Experiencing difficulties when trying to fully extend the hip, which can make activities such as walking, running, and climbing stairs more demanding.

A noticeable sensation of stiffness in the hip area, particularly after extended periods of inactivity.

> **Postural Problems:**

Anterior Pelvic Tilt: Tight hip flexors can result in a forward tilt of the pelvis, which can lead to an excessive curve in the lower back and compromised posture.

Compensatory Movements: The body may develop alternative movement patterns to alleviate discomfort, which can result in additional musculoskeletal imbalances and potential injuries.

> **Effects on Physical Activities:**

Optimal athletic performance can be hindered by tight hip flexors, leading to a decrease in power and efficiency during sports activities. This can have a negative impact on running, jumping, and other dynamic movements.

Restrictions on Physical Activity: Experiencing challenges with exercises that involve hip extension or flexion, such as lunges, squats, and leg lifts.

> **Everyday limitations in functionality:**

Challenging Getting on Your Feet: Transitioning from a seated position can often be a difficult and uncomfortable task.

Walking and running can be uncomfortable and inefficient due to pain and reduced range of motion.

Comfort during sitting can be compromised by the pressure exerted on tight hip flexors over time.

Gaining a comprehensive understanding of the typical triggers of tight hip flexors and the associated symptoms is the initial stride in effectively tackling this matter. Through an understanding of the effects on daily life, you can implement proactive measures like integrating regular stretching, strengthening exercises, and making lifestyle adjustments to relieve tightness and enhance overall hip health.

CHAPTER TWO

Identifying Tight Hip Flexors

Simple Tests to Identify Tightness

Identifying tight hip flexors is the initial step in addressing the problem. Here are a few straightforward tests you can do at home to evaluate the flexibility of your hip flexors:

- ➢ **Thomas Test:**

Position yourself on a horizontal surface, lying on your back. Bring one knee towards your chest, grasping it with your hands. Allow the opposite leg to rest and stretch beyond the surface.

The extended leg lifting off the surface or a sensation of stretching in the front of the hip may suggest tightness in the hip flexors.

> **Testing the Kneeling Hip Flexor Stretch:**

Assume a kneeling position with one knee on the ground and the other foot positioned in front, creating a 90-degree angle at both knees. Make sure to maintain a straight back as you gently move your hips forward.

Based on observations, individuals may experience a notable stretch in the hip of the kneeling leg or encounter challenges when attempting to push their hips forward, which could indicate tightness in the hip flexors.

> ### **Test for Straight Leg Raise:**

Assume a supine position with both legs fully extended. Elevate one leg to its maximum height while ensuring the other leg remains parallel to the ground.

If the leg cannot reach a 90-degree angle with the body or if there is a sensation of tightness in the hip, it may indicate tight hip flexors.

> ### **Butterfly Stretch Examination:**

Assume a seated position on the floor, ensuring that your feet are together, and your knees are bent outwards. Focus on applying pressure to your knees with your elbows, aiming to bring them closer to the floor.

If you are feeling any discomfort or are unable to bring your knees close to the floor, it could be a sign of tightness in your hip flexors or inner thigh muscles.

Exploring Your Range of Motion

Understanding your hip range of motion can provide valuable insights into the level of tightness in your hip flexors. Here's a method to evaluate it:

➢ **Examining hip flexion:**

Assume a supine position with your legs extended. Raise one leg towards your chest, maintaining a bent knee.

Optimal Range: It is ideal to have the ability to bring your thigh close to your torso, resulting in a hip angle of at least 120 degrees.

➢ **Extension of the hip:**

Position yourself in a prone position on a level surface. Raise one leg off the ground while keeping it extended.

It is expected that you are able to lift your leg to create a minimum angle of 10-15 degrees from the ground.

➢ **Hip Abduction:**

Position yourself on your side, ensuring that your bottom leg is bent to provide stability. Raise the upper leg in a vertical direction towards the ceiling.

It is expected that you are able to lift your leg to a minimum of a 45-degree angle.

Examination of hip adduction:

Position yourself on your side, with the upper leg bent and crossed over the lower leg. Raise the lower leg towards the ceiling.

Expected Range: It is expected that you can lift your leg to a minimum of a 30-degree angle.

Examining Hip Internal and External Rotation:

Take a seat on a chair and ensure that your knees are bent at a 90-degree angle. Examine the movement of your foot as you rotate it both inward and outward from the knee.

It is expected that you have the ability to rotate your hip internally and externally to approximately a 45-degree angle.

When to Consider Professional Assistance

Although self-care and exercise can often help with tight hip flexors, there are instances where seeking professional assistance becomes essential. Here's a guide to help you determine when it may be beneficial to seek advice from a healthcare professional:

➢ **Chronic and Persistent Pain:**

If you're dealing with persistent pain in your hips, lower back, or thighs that doesn't seem to get better with stretching and exercise, it may be a good idea to consult with a professional.

➢ **Intense Tightness:**

If your hip flexors are causing significant limitations in your range of motion or daily activities, it may be necessary to seek professional intervention.

> **Injury or Trauma:**

If you have experienced an injury or trauma to your hip area, such as a fall or direct impact, and are currently dealing with pain or tightness, it is advisable to seek medical attention.

> **Swelling or inflammation:**

If you observe any swelling, redness, or warmth around your hip area, it may suggest the presence of inflammation or an underlying condition that should be assessed by a professional.

> **Sensation of Numbness or Tingling:**

If you notice any numbness, tingling, or weakness in your legs or hips, it is important to have it evaluated by a healthcare provider as it may indicate nerve involvement.

> **Challenges with Mobility:**

If you're experiencing difficulty with walking, standing, or completing daily activities because of hip tightness or pain, it's crucial to seek a professional evaluation.

By conducting basic tests, you can easily pinpoint any issues with your hip flexors and gain insight into the extent of your mobility. Nevertheless, if you encounter long-lasting or severe symptoms, it is essential to seek assistance from a professional. A healthcare provider can provide a thorough assessment and customized treatment plan to meet your individual requirements, guaranteeing the restoration of your hip's optimal function and mobility.

Impact of Tight Hip Flexors on Posture

The impact of tight hip flexors on posture can be significant, as they are attached to key points and play a crucial role in stabilizing the pelvis and spine. This is how they impact posture:

> **Anterior Pelvic Tilt:**

Tight hip flexors, particularly the iliopsoas, result in the pelvis being pulled forward and downward, leading to an anterior pelvic tilt.

This tilt leads to an increased lumbar curve (lordosis), causing the lower back to arch excessively. In addition, it may result in a noticeable protrusion of the abdomen and a decrease in the appearance of the glutes.

➤ Lumbar Spine Stress:

The anterior pelvic tilt results in an increased lumbar lordosis, which places added strain on the lumbar spine.

Over time, the body's posture can result in muscle imbalances, discomfort, and potential degenerative changes in the spine. This is caused by the abnormal curvature and stress distribution.

➤ Upper Body Alignment:

When the pelvis tilts forward, it has an impact on the alignment of the entire upper body.

Due to the pelvic tilt, the upper body may lean backward, resulting in a misalignment that can impact the neck, shoulders, and overall posture.

➢ **Hip and Knee Alignment:**

The alignment of the hips and knees can be affected by tight hip flexors.

The misalignment can lead to knee hyperextension and outward foot rotation, which can have a significant impact on both posture and gait.

CHAPTER THREE

Effects on Mobility and Athletic Performance

Tight hip flexors can have a considerable impact on both mobility and athletic performance. Here's the step-by-step process:

> **Restricted Range of Motion:**

Restricted hip flexors can impede the complete extension of the hip joint. Restrictions on mobility can pose challenges when it comes to engaging in activities that demand a wide range of motion, like running, jumping, and squatting. Movements exhibit a decrease in fluidity and an increase in restriction.

> **Impaired Athletic Performance:**

Numerous athletic activities require a high degree of hip mobility. The effects of tight hip flexors include a reduction in stride length during running, a decrease in power and speed while sprinting, and an impairment in the ability to jump high or change directions quickly. Athletes may experience difficulties in generating force from the hips, which can have an impact on their overall performance.

> **High Risk of injury.**

Tight hip flexors can lead to muscle imbalances and affect biomechanics. These imbalances may result in the overuse of other muscles, which can heighten the likelihood of injuries like strains, sprains, and even stress fractures. Understanding the importance of proper hip flexor function is essential for maintaining balance and stability during athletic activities.

> **Tiredness and excessive use:**

Having tight hip flexors can result in muscle fatigue occurring earlier than expected. Athletes may experience quicker fatigue as a result of other muscles having to exert more effort in order to compensate for the tightness in their hip flexors. These factors can lead to a decrease in endurance and an increased risk of overuse injuries.

Link Between Lower Back Pain and Other Health Problems

Extensive research has established a clear link between tight hip flexors and lower back pain. Understanding the connection between tight hip flexors and various issues, such as back pain, is crucial.

> ## Compression of the lumbar spine:

Tight hip flexors can lead to a forward tilt of the pelvis, which in turn can result in an increased curvature of the lumbar spine. The increased curvature of the spine places extra pressure on the lumbar vertebrae and intervertebral discs, resulting in discomfort in the lower back. Over time, this can lead to the development of conditions like disc herniation or degenerative disc disease.

> ## Muscle Imbalances:

Tight hip flexors are commonly found alongside weak glutes and hamstrings, resulting in an imbalance. The imbalance in the body causes the lower back muscles to work harder than they should, resulting in muscle strain and discomfort. Chronic lower back discomfort can arise from the body's efforts to stabilize the pelvis and spine through tight hip flexors.

> **Altered Patterns of Movement:**

Individuals may modify their movement patterns to alleviate discomfort or address stiffness. These changed patterns can cause strain on other areas of the body, like the knees and ankles, which may result in further injuries and discomfort. Over time, these repetitive movements can lead to long-term problems.

> **Referred Pain:**

Tight hip flexors can lead to pain in other areas of the body. The pain can extend to the buttocks, thighs, or even down to the knees, resembling conditions such as sciatica. Understanding the hip flexors' role as the underlying factor is crucial for successful treatment.

> ### ➢ **Pelvic Floor Dysfunction:**

The iliopsoas muscle is closely connected to the pelvic floor muscles. The effects of tight hip flexors can contribute to pelvic floor dysfunction, resulting in symptoms like pelvic pain, urinary incontinence, and other related issues in the pelvic area.

Having tight hip flexors can have a significant impact on your posture, mobility, and athletic performance. It can also contribute to lower back pain and other related issues. Gaining insight into these connections emphasizes the significance of consistently engaging in stretching, strengthening exercises, and mindful movement to maintain flexible and strong hip flexors. By being proactive in addressing tight hip flexors, you can experience benefits such as improved posture, enhanced athletic performance, and a decrease in pain and discomfort.

Types and Advantages of Stretching

Stretching provides a wide range of advantages that go beyond just enhancing flexibility. Provided is a comprehensive summary of the physiological and mental/emotional advantages of stretching:

> **Physiological Advantages**

1. Enhanced Flexibility:

Through regular stretching, the length and elasticity of muscles and connective tissues can be increased, leading to improved flexibility. Greater flexibility improves your range of motion, making everyday activities and physical exercises easier and more efficient.

2. Improved Muscle Performance:

Stretching enhances muscle function by optimizing the way muscles and tendons work together. Enhancing overall physical performance by improving strength, speed, and endurance.

3. Decreased Risk of Injury:

Stretching enhances the flexibility and durability of muscles and joints. Stretching has numerous benefits as it helps in preparing muscles for physical activity, thus reducing the risk of strains, sprains, and other injuries.

4. Enhanced Posture:

Stretching helps to address muscle imbalances and elongate tight muscles that can lead to suboptimal posture. Improved posture can help alleviate strain on your spine and the muscles surrounding it, which can lead to a reduction in pain and discomfort.

5. Improved Circulation:

Stretching helps to increase blood flow to muscles and joints. Improved circulation enhances the delivery of oxygen and nutrients to muscle tissues, promoting faster recovery and reducing muscle soreness by eliminating metabolic waste.

6. Decreased Muscle Tension and Pain:

Stretching aids in the release of muscle tightness and knots. It effectively relieves discomfort and pain, especially in areas that are often tense, such as the neck, shoulders, and lower back.

7. Enhanced Range of Motion:

Stretching aids in preserving and expanding the range of motion in your joints. The increased range of motion provided by this product allows for easier completion of everyday tasks and participation in physical activities, reducing the likelihood of sustaining injuries.

8. Prevention of Muscle Imbalances:

Stretching aids in maintaining a harmonious muscle length and function. Having well-balanced muscles can help minimize the chances of experiencing overuse injuries and improve your overall movement patterns.

➢ **Benefits for the Mind and Emotions**

1. Stress Relief:

Stretching encourages relaxation and helps decrease the release of stress hormones such as cortisol. It aids in relieving physical and mental tension, offering a feeling of tranquility and relaxation.

2. Enhanced Mood:

Stretching has the potential to stimulate the release of endorphins, which are natural mood enhancers in the body. Regular stretching has been found to have numerous benefits, including improving mood, reducing anxiety, and enhancing emotional well-being.

3. Mindfulness and Relaxation:

Stretching promotes a sense of mindfulness by directing your attention to your body and breath. This mindfulness practice can assist in reducing mental stress and fostering a state of relaxation and mindfulness in the present moment.

4. Improved Mental Clarity:

Stretching can enhance cognitive function by improving blood flow to the brain and reducing physical tension. Improved focus, concentration, and mental clarity are crucial for daily activities and decision-making.

5. Improved Sleep:

Incorporating stretching into your bedtime routine can promote relaxation of both your body and mind, facilitating a more restful and uninterrupted sleep. Improved sleep quality has a positive impact on overall health, mood, and cognitive function.

6. Enhanced Body Awareness:

Stretching aids in developing a heightened sense of your body's sensations and movements. Increased body awareness can lead to improvements in coordination, balance, and overall physical performance.

7. Reduction of Symptoms in Mental Health Conditions:

Stretching, especially when combined with deep breathing or yoga practices, has been found to have a positive impact on symptoms of depression and anxiety. It can be used as an additional method to traditional mental health treatments, aiding in the management and relief of symptoms.

Integrating regular stretching into your routine provides a broad spectrum of physiological and mental/emotional advantages. Stretching offers a wide range of benefits, including increased flexibility and performance, decreased stress levels, and a better mood. It is a straightforward yet impactful practice that promotes overall well-being. Through a thorough understanding and firsthand experience of these advantages, incorporating stretching into your health and fitness routine can become a consistent and valuable practice.

Various Forms of Stretching

Stretching can be classified into various types, each with distinct techniques and advantages. Provided is a comprehensive overview of the most prevalent types of stretching.

- Static stretching,

- Dynamic stretching,

- PNF (Proprioceptive Neuromuscular Facilitation)

- **Static Stretching:**

Static stretching requires maintaining a stretch for a prolonged duration, usually ranging from 15 to 60 seconds, without any movement. The main emphasis is on extending the muscle to its maximum extent and maintaining the position.

Advantages:

Static stretching can enhance flexibility by maintaining the muscle in a stretched position.

• Improves Muscle Relaxation: Maintaining a stretch can aid in muscle relaxation and the release of tension.

• Regular static stretching can enhance muscle elasticity, potentially reducing the risk of injuries.

• Static stretching after exercise can aid in recovery by reducing muscle stiffness and soreness.

Here are some examples:

- **Hamstring Stretch:** Perform the hamstring stretch by sitting on the ground with one leg extended and the other bent. Extend your leg and grasp your toes, maintaining the position.

- **Quadriceps Stretch:** Perform the quadriceps stretch by standing on one leg, pulling the other foot towards the glutes, and maintaining the position.

- **Calf Stretch:** Perform the calf stretch by positioning one foot forward and the other foot back. Apply pressure to the back heel as you lean forward, effectively stretching the calf.

➤ **Dynamic Stretching:**

Dynamic stretching entails actively moving different parts of your body through a complete range of motion in a controlled manner. These stretches are commonly done prior to physical activity to prime the muscles for exercise.

Advantages:

• Dynamic stretching is effective in raising the heart rate and improving blood flow to the muscles, which helps to warm them up for activity.

• Dynamic stretching is known to enhance athletic performance by replicating the movements of the activity you are about to engage in. This can lead to improved performance and better results.

• Dynamic stretches are great for improving the functional range of motion. They work by engaging multiple muscle groups and joints, which helps enhance functional flexibility and coordination.

•Warming up with dynamic stretching can help minimize the risk of injury by preparing the body for physical activity.

Here are some examples:

- Perform leg swings by standing on one leg and swinging the other leg in different directions - forward and backward, as well as side to side.

- Perform arm circles by extending your arms to the sides and making small to large circles in both directions.

- Perform walking lunges by stepping forward into a lunge and alternating legs as you move forward.

➢ **PNF (Proprioceptive Neuromuscular Facilitation)**

This is a stretching technique that combines both stretching and contracting the specific muscle group. Typically, a partner or prop is needed for this activity, which focuses on a sequence of contractions and relaxations to enhance flexibility.

Advantages:

- **Enhances Flexibility:** PNF is renowned for its effectiveness in improving static-passive flexibility.

- **Enhances Muscle Strength:** The contract-relax techniques can also contribute to the improvement of muscle strength.

PNF stretching has been found to greatly enhance the range of motion in joints.

- **Enhances Muscle Coordination:** Through the combination of stretching and isometric contractions, PNF can improve neuromuscular coordination.

Method:

- **Hold-Relax:** Extend the muscle to its maximum capacity and maintain the position for a brief period, then exert force against resistance for 5-10 seconds, followed by a more intense stretch.

• **Contract-Relax:** Similar to hold-relax, but the contraction is performed by moving through the range of motion against resistance.

• **Contract-Relax-Agonist-Contract (CRAC):** Following the hold-relax phase, the antagonist muscle group is contracted to further enhance the stretch.

Here are some examples:

• **Hamstring PNF Stretch:** Assume a supine position and elevate one leg. Engage in a collaborative exercise where your leg is gently pushed towards you by a partner, prompting you to resist the force. Afterward, allow yourself to relax and permit your partner to push your leg even further.

• **Shoulder PNF Stretch:** Stand facing a wall and place your forearm against it. Push against the wall while engaging your shoulder muscles, then relax and stretch a bit further.

Gaining a comprehensive understanding of the various types of stretching and the advantages they offer enables you to seamlessly integrate them into your fitness regimen. Static stretching is recommended for post-workout recovery and improving flexibility. Dynamic stretching is more suitable for pre-workout warm-ups and enhancing performance. PNF stretching is known for its ability to greatly increase flexibility and muscle coordination. Through the incorporation of these stretching techniques, one can enhance their overall physical performance, minimize the likelihood of injury, and optimize muscle health.

CHAPTER FOUR

Effective Stretching Routines for Maximum Results

Integrating stretching routines into your daily routine can have a substantial impact on your flexibility, muscle tension, and overall well-being. Here are some precise routines and focused stretching exercises to assist you in attaining these advantages.

➢ **Everyday Stretching Routine**

Neck Stretch:

Maintain an upright posture while sitting or standing. Slowly tilt your head to the right, bringing your ear towards your shoulder. Hold for 15-30 seconds and then switch to the other side. Perform 2-3 repetitions on each side.

- **Shoulder Stretch:**

Cross one arm over your chest and grasp it with the hand on the opposite side. Ensure that your shoulders remain in a relaxed position. Hold for 15-30 seconds, then switch sides. Perform 2-3 repetitions on each side.

- **The Cat-Cow Stretch:**

Begin by positioning yourself on all fours. Curve your back (cow pose) and then flex it (cat pose). Transition seamlessly between the positions. Repeat for 10-12 cycles.

- **Standing Hamstring Stretch:**

Begin by positioning your feet about hip-width apart. Lean forward at the hips, maintaining a straight back, and extend your arms towards your toes. Maintain for 15-30 seconds.

- **Stretching the quadriceps muscles:**

Balance on a single leg while bringing the foot of the other leg towards your glutes. Ensure that your knees are positioned in close proximity to each other. Maintain each side for 15-30 seconds.

- **The Calf Stretch exercise:**

Position yourself in front of a wall. Position one foot behind, firmly plant the heel into the ground, and incline the body forward. Maintain each side for 15-30 seconds.

> ➢ **Morning Stretches for Hip Flexors**

- **Hip Flexor Lunge:**

Begin by assuming a lunge position, with one foot positioned forward and the other knee resting on the ground. Move your hips forward with caution. Maintain each side for 20-30 seconds without interruption.

- **Butterfly Stretch:**

Assume a seated position with your feet touching and your knees angled outward. Ensure that you apply a gentle pressure to your knees, directing them towards the floor. Maintain for 20-30 seconds.

- **The Standing Hip Flexor Stretch:**

Position yourself with one foot in front and the other behind. Flex the front knee while maintaining a straight back leg and propel your hips forward. Maintain each side for 20-30 seconds without interruption.

- **Knee-to-Chest Stretch:**

Lie on your back and bring one knee towards your chest, securely holding it with both hands. Maintain the other leg in a straight position. Maintain each side for 20-30 seconds without interruption.

- ➢ **Evening Stretches for Enhanced Flexibility**

- **Forward Bend:**

Assume a standing position with feet close together, gently lean forward at the hips, and allow the upper body to dangle downwards. Extend your arms downwards and try to touch your toes or the floor. Maintain for 30-60 seconds.

- **Child's Pose:**

Begin by positioning yourself on all fours, then gradually shift your weight back onto your heels. Simultaneously, reach your arms forward and gradually lower your chest towards the ground. Maintain for 30-60 seconds.

- **Pigeon Pose:**

Starting from a plank position, carefully bring one knee forward and position it behind your wrist. Extend the other leg behind you and gradually lower your hips. Maintain each side for 30-60 seconds without interruption.

- **Seated Forward Fold:**

Assume a seated position with your legs fully extended in front of you. Extend your arms towards your toes, ensuring that your back remains in proper alignment. Maintain for 30-60 seconds.

> **Effective Stretching Exercises for Specific Areas**

- **Butterfly Stretch**

Assume a seated position with your feet touching and your knees angled outward. Ensure that you apply a gentle pressure to your knees, directing them towards the floor. Targets and stretches the muscles in the inner thighs, groin, and hips. Maintain for 20-30 seconds.

- **Pigeon Pose:**

Starting from a plank position, carefully bring one knee forward and position it behind your wrist. Extend the other leg behind you and gradually lower your hips.

This exercise targets and stretches the hip flexors, glutes, and lower back. Maintain the position for 30-60 seconds on each side.

- **Hip Flexor Lunge:**

Begin by assuming a lunge position, with one foot positioned forward and the other knee resting on the ground. Ensure that you gently push your hips forward. This exercise helps to elongate and strengthen the muscles in the hip flexors and quadriceps. Maintain each side for 20-30 seconds without interruption.

- **Frog Stretch:**

Begin by positioning yourself on all fours, with your knees spread apart and your hips gradually descending towards the ground.

Ensure that your feet remain aligned with your knees throughout the movement. Targets and stretches the muscles in the inner thighs, groin, and hips. Maintain for 30-60 seconds.

By integrating these stretching routines into your daily routine, you can effectively preserve your flexibility, alleviate muscle tension, and enhance your overall physical and mental well-being. By incorporating morning stretches, evening flexibility exercises, and targeted routines for areas like the hip flexors, you can work towards achieving a healthier and more balanced body.

Strengthening Exercises

Strengthening exercises are a valuable addition to stretching routines as they help maintain muscle flexibility, strength, and balance. This combination is effective in maintaining optimal muscle function, enhancing posture, and minimizing the risk of injuries. Here's how stretching helps to prevent the reoccurrence of tightness:

- **Ensuring Well-Rounded Muscle Growth:**

Stretching helps to lengthen muscles, which can enhance flexibility. Strengthening exercises help develop muscle strength, which is crucial for ensuring that muscles can effectively support joints. This equilibrium aids in preventing muscle imbalances that may result in tightness and potential injury.

- **Enhanced Posture and Alignment:**

Developing the core, back, and other stabilizing muscles is crucial for maintaining correct posture and spinal alignment. Having proper posture is essential for minimizing strain on your muscles and joints, which can help prevent the reoccurrence of tightness, particularly in areas such as the hip flexors and lower back.

- **Improved Muscle Performance:**

Efficient muscles are able to work more effectively, making daily activities and exercise require less effort. Optimizing muscle function can help minimize the risk of overuse and the resulting tightness and discomfort.

- **Preventing Injuries:**

By focusing on strengthening muscles and improving flexibility, the chances of experiencing strains, sprains, and other injuries can be significantly reduced. Ensuring a comprehensive fitness routine that incorporates both stretching and strengthening exercises can provide enhanced protection for muscles and joints during physical activity.

- **Enhanced Stability and Mobility:**

Strengthening exercises help to enhance joint stability, while stretching can improve mobility. This combination ensures that joints move smoothly through their entire range of motion, minimizing the risk of tightness and injury.

Efficient Strengthening Exercises

By integrating targeted strengthening exercises into your routine, you can effectively preserve flexibility and proactively ward off tightness. These exercises have been proven to be effective:

- **Glute Bridges Method:**

Assume a supine position with your knees flexed and feet resting flat on the floor, maintaining a distance equal to the width of your hips.

Focus on driving power from your heels as you raise your hips towards the ceiling, engaging your glutes at the peak of the movement. Then return your hips to the starting position. Perform 3 sets of 12-15 repetitions.

Advantages:

- Enhances the strength of the glutes, lower back, and core.

- Enhances hip stability and alleviates tension in the hip flexors.

- **Leg Raises Method:**

Assume a supine position with your legs extended. Ensure that your hands remain at your sides or beneath your lower back to provide support. Raise your legs towards the ceiling, ensuring they remain straight.

Gently lower them down to the initial position, making sure not to make contact with the floor. Perform 3 sets of 10-12 repetitions.

Advantages:

- Enhances the strength of the lower abdominal muscles and hip flexors.

- Enhances core stability and alleviates tension in the lower back and hips.

Effective Core Strengthening Exercises

> **Plank:**

Begin by assuming a push-up position, ensuring that your body forms a straight line from your head to your heels. Stay in your current position. Hold for 30-60 seconds. Perform the task 2-3 times. It enhances the strength of the core, shoulders, and lower back. Improves overall stability and posture.

> **Russian Twists:**

Assume a seated position on the floor, with your knees bent and feet resting flat on the ground. Lean back slightly and grasp a weight or medicine ball. Rotate your torso in one direction, and then in the opposite direction. Hold for 30-60 seconds. Perform the task 2-3 times. It Enhances the strength of the oblique muscles and enhances rotational stability.

> **Bird-Dog:**

Begin by positioning yourself on all fours. Reach your right arm forward and extend your left leg back, maintaining stability in your body. Go back to the initial position and change sides. Perform 3 sets of 10-12 repetitions on each side.

It enhances the strength of the core, lower back, and glutes. Enhances balance and coordination.

Exercises with Resistance Bands

> **Clamshells:**

Position a resistance band around your thighs, slightly above your knees. Assume a position where you are lying on your side with your knees bent at a 90-degree angle.

Raise your upper knee while maintaining the position of your feet, then proceed to lower it. Perform 3 sets of 15-20 repetitions on each side. It enhances the strength of the glutes and hip abductors. Enhances hip stability and alleviates tightness.

> ➢ **Band Walks:**

Secure a resistance band around your ankles. Assume a stance with your feet positioned hip-width apart and a slight bend in your knees. Take a step to the side with one foot, and then follow with the other, ensuring that you maintain tension in the band. It enhances the strength of the glutes, hips, and thighs. Enhances lateral hip stability and alleviates any tightness. Perform 3 sets of 10-12 steps on each side.

> ➢ **Banded Hip Thrusts:**

Position a resistance band around your thighs, slightly above your knees. Position yourself on the ground, ensuring your upper back is resting against a bench and your feet are firmly planted on the floor. Focus on driving power from your heels as you raise your hips towards the ceiling, engaging your glutes at the peak of the movement. It enhances the strength of the glutes, hamstrings, and lower back. Improves hip stability and alleviates tightness. Perform 3 sets of 12-15 repetitions.

It is essential to incorporate both stretching and strengthening exercises into your routine in order to maintain flexibility, prevent muscle tightness, and promote overall muscle health. Integrate these highly effective strengthening exercises into your routine to enhance your stretching efforts, enhance posture, and minimize the likelihood of injury. Through a careful and systematic approach to fitness, one can attain a body that is both healthier and more resilient.

CHAPTER FIVE

Understanding Myofascial Release

MFR is a form of therapy that effectively alleviates tension and pain in the body's myofascial tissues. These tough membranes play a crucial role in wrapping, connecting, and supporting your muscles. The objective is to eliminate limitations in the myofascial tissues in order to regain mobility and relieve discomfort.

Fascia is a vital component of the body's structure, enveloping muscles, bones, and joints to offer essential support and safeguarding.

Myofascial restrictions happen when fascia becomes tight or constricted because of injury, stress, or poor posture, resulting in pain and restricted mobility.

Advantages of MFR:

- Increased flexibility,

- Decreased muscle soreness,

- Improved blood flow, and

- Reduced pain and stiffness.

Foam Rolling Techniques for Hip Flexors

Using a cylindrical foam roller, foam rolling is a widely practiced method of myofascial release that applies pressure to areas of tightness or discomfort.

➢ **Hip Flexors Foam Roll:**

Begin by lying face down on the floor and placing the foam roller under your hip flexors. Perform the action by gently moving back and forth from just below your hip bone to the top of your thigh. Take a moment to focus on any areas that feel tight or sore. Allocate 1-2 minutes for each side.

➢ **Quadriceps Foam Roll:**

Assume a prone position with the foam roller positioned beneath your thighs.

Perform the movement by smoothly transitioning from your hip to the area just above your knee, with a specific emphasis on targeting the muscles at the front of your thighs. Take a moment to focus on any areas that feel particularly tense or constricted. Allocate 1-2 minutes for each leg.

> **Iliotibial (IT) Band Foam Roll:**

Assume a side-lying position with the foam roller positioned beneath your outer thigh. Perform a rolling motion from your hip to just above your knee, with emphasis on the side of your thigh. This can have an indirect impact on the hip flexors. Allocate 1-2 minutes for each side.

Techniques for Self-Massage

Self-massage is a highly effective method for relieving muscle and fascia tension, eliminating the need for a foam roller.

➢ **Releasing the Hip Flexors:**

Assume a supine position with your knees flexed. Apply gentle pressure to your hip flexors, just below your hip bones, using your fingers or a massage ball. Massage the area by moving in small circles. Allocate 1-2 minutes for each side.

➢ **Massage for the Thigh:**

Find a relaxed and cozy position to sit or lie down. Employ your hands or a massage tool to manipulate your thigh muscles, commencing at the knee and progressing towards the hip. Apply consistent and controlled force. Allocate 1-2 minutes for each leg.

> **Massage for the Lower Back:**

Begin by lying on your back with your knees bent. Apply gentle pressure to the muscles on either side of your spine using your fingers or a massage ball. Performing circular motions can help alleviate tension. Allocate 1-2 minutes for each side.

Self-Massage Tools

There are a variety of tools available that can help improve your self-massage routine, allowing you to effectively apply pressure to specific areas.

> **Foam Rollers:**

These cylindrical foam tools are designed to effectively apply pressure to large muscle groups. Great for targeting the hip flexors, quads, IT band, and other major muscle groups.

> **Massage Balls:**

These small, firm balls (such as tennis balls or lacrosse balls) are designed to apply precise pressure. Beneficial for targeting and relieving tension in the hip flexors, lower back, and other areas that are typically difficult to access.

> **Massage Sticks:**

These handheld sticks with rollers are designed to target and apply pressure to specific muscles. Ideal for performing self-massage on the thighs, calves, and other areas that are easily reachable.

➤ **Percussion Massagers:**

Electric devices that provide quick and repetitive muscle stimulation. Great for deep tissue massage and myofascial release.

Step-by-Step Guide to Self-Massage Preparation:

- Find a cozy environment: Select a serene and cozy space where you can unwind.

- Prepare: Begin your workout by engaging in light physical activity or stretching to warm up your muscles.

- Identify Tight Areas:

Utilize your tactile senses to identify any areas of tension or discomfort within your muscles. Areas of focus commonly include the hip flexors, thighs, and lower back.

- Apply Pressure:

Apply pressure to the tight area using your fingers, hands, or a massage tool. Begin with a gentle touch and gradually apply more force as necessary. Employ deliberate, methodical movements or utilize a pressing technique to alleviate the strain.

- Hold and Release:

In the event that you come across a particularly tense area, maintain the pressure for a duration of 20-30 seconds until you sense the muscle loosening. Take deep breaths to promote muscle relaxation.

- Expand the Area:

Following the massage, carefully elongate the muscle to promote improved circulation and enhanced flexibility. After giving your hip flexors a nice massage, it's a good idea to follow up with a hip flexor stretch.

- Stay properly hydrated:

Remember to drink an ample amount of water after your self-massage session. This will aid in eliminating any toxins that may have been released and will also keep your muscles well-hydrated.

Using techniques such as foam rolling and self-massage, myofascial release can effectively alleviate muscle tension and enhance flexibility. By incorporating these practices into your routine and utilizing suitable tools, one can effectively maintain healthy and relaxed muscles, thus preventing any potential tightness. By following the step-by-step guide, you can ensure an effective self-massage and experience the numerous benefits it has to offer.

Yoga Poses for Relieving Tension in the Hip Flexors

Yoga is a highly effective practice for relieving tension in the hip flexors, enhancing flexibility, and fostering a sense of overall well-being. By integrating certain yoga poses into your routine, you can effectively address tightness in the hip flexors and improve overall mobility.

Best yoga poses for hip flexor health.

➢ **Low Lunge**

Begin by assuming a high lunge stance, with your right foot positioned forward and your left knee resting on the ground. Shift your hips forward and downward, experiencing a gentle stretch in your left hip flexor, raise your arms above your head and maintain the position. This exercise targets and stretches key muscles in the hips and thighs. Hold for 30-60 seconds on each side, taking into account the appropriate duration for optimal results.

> **Pigeon Pose**

Pigeon Pose is a yoga posture that provides a deep stretch and release for the hips and lower back. It is a pose that requires focus and attention to detail in order to achieve proper alignment and maximize its benefits.

Begin in a tabletop position and carefully move your right knee forward, positioning it behind your right wrist. Extend your left leg straight back and lower your hips towards the ground. Lean forward and place your forehead on the mat or a block.

It enhances hip mobility, elongates the muscles in the hips, buttocks, and lower back. Hold for 1-2 minutes on each side.

> **Warrior I**

Begin by assuming a standing position, then proceed to step your right foot forward into a lunge. Simultaneously, rotate your left foot outward at a 45-degree angle. Flex your right knee and raise your arms above your head. Ensure that your hips remain parallel and focus on the sensation of the stretch in your left hip flexor. This exercise targets the hip flexors, enhances leg strength, and enhances balance. Hold for 30-60 seconds on each side.

> **Bridge Pose**

Assume a supine position with your knees flexed and feet positioned at a distance equal to the width of your hips. Rise up by pushing through your feet, elevating your hips towards the ceiling while engaging your glutes. Ensure that your arms remain by your sides or securely clasped under your back. It enhances the strength of the glutes and lower back while also providing a gentle stretch to the hip flexors. Hold for 30-60 seconds.

> **Butterfly Pose**

Assume a seated position with your feet touching and your knees angled outward. Grasp your feet with your hands and apply a gentle pressure to encourage your knees to move closer to the floor. This exercise targets and elongates the muscles in the inner thighs, groin, and hip flexors. Hold for 1-2 minutes.

Maintaining a Regular Yoga Practice

- Practicing yoga 3-5 times per week can lead to noticeable improvements in flexibility and hip health. Start with a gentle warm-up, like Sun Salutations, to get your muscles ready for more intense stretches.

- Be mindful of the signals your body is sending and refrain from pushing yourself beyond your limits. Adjust poses as necessary.

- Emphasize the importance of deep, mindful breathing during your practice to promote relaxation and alleviate tension.

Strengthen Your Hip Flexors with Pilates

Pilates is a highly effective method for strengthening and stretching the hip flexors, which helps improve balance and core stability.

- ➢ **Single Leg Stretch.**

Position yourself by lying on your back with your knees bent and feet flat on the floor. Raise your head, neck, and shoulders from the mat and draw your right knee towards your chest as you lengthen your left leg. Alternate the movement of your legs in a scissoring motion. It enhances the strength of the core, hip flexors, and quads. Perform 10-15 repetitions per leg.

- ➢ **Leg Circles:**

Lie on your back with your arms resting by your sides and your legs fully extended. Raise your right leg towards the ceiling and rotate it in small circles. Change the direction after completing a few circles. It enhances hip mobility and fortifies the hip flexors and core, resulting in numerous benefits. Perform 5-10 circles in each direction per leg.

> **Hundred:**

Position yourself by lying on your back with your knees bent and feet flat on the floor. Raise your head, neck, and shoulders off the mat and stretch out your legs to a 45-degree angle. Ensure that you maintain a consistent arm motion while synchronizing your breath, inhaling and exhaling for five counts each. It enhances core strength, hip flexor function, and boosts cardiovascular endurance. Perform 10 sets of 10 pumps.

Benefits of Pilates for Flexibility and Strength

> **Enhanced Flexibility:**

Pilates focuses on precise movements and stretches that improve flexibility in the muscles and joints, with a particular emphasis on the hips and lower back.

Regular practice of this activity can result in an expansion of your range of motion and a decrease in muscle stiffness.

> **Strength at the core:**

Pilates places a strong emphasis on core engagement, which plays a crucial role in stabilizing and providing support to the lower back and hips.

One of the advantages of having a strong core is that it helps to minimize the chances of sustaining injuries and enhances your posture and balance.

> **Muscle Tone and Strength:**

Pilates exercises focus on engaging various muscle groups, ensuring a well-rounded and balanced muscle development. Strengthening the hip flexors, glutes, and other stabilizing muscles can help prevent tightness and improve functional movement.

> **Mind-Body Connection:**

Pilates promotes a thoughtful approach to movement and emphasizes the importance of controlling your breath, which helps develop a heightened understanding of how your body works. This increased awareness can enhance movement patterns and help avoid excessive or incorrect use of muscles.

Integrating yoga and Pilates into your regular routine can greatly enhance the health of your hip flexors. These practices work to improve flexibility, strength, and overall body awareness, leading to significant benefits for your hip flexors. Consistent practice of specific poses and exercises can aid in the release of tension, the prevention of tightness, and the promotion of a well-balanced, healthy body. Through a comprehensive understanding of the advantages and methods of both disciplines, one can develop a holistic fitness routine that promotes optimal hip flexor function and overall wellness.

CHAPTER SIX

Ergonomics and Posture

Maintaining correct ergonomics and posture is critical for avoiding musculoskeletal issues, minimizing discomfort, and increasing productivity. Understanding how to create an ergonomic office and practice excellent posture can dramatically improve your general health and well-being.

Setting Up an Ergonomic Workspace

Creating an ergonomic workspace entails arranging office equipment and furnishings to meet your body's needs and promote proper posture.

Chair:

Adjustable Seat Height: Position your feet flat on the floor and your knees at a 90-degree angle.

Lumbar Support: To keep your spine's natural curve, use a chair that provides adequate lower back support.

Adjust the armrests so that your elbows form a 90-degree angle and your shoulders relax.

Desk:

Your desk should be set at a height where your forearms are parallel to the floor while typing.

Clearance: Make sure there is enough space beneath the desk for your legs to move comfortably.

Monitor:

Height and Distance: Place the display at eye level, approximately an arm's length away. The top of the screen should be at or slightly below eye level.

Glare: Adjust the screen to reduce glare from windows or overhead lights.

Keyboard and Mouse:

Placement: Keep the keyboard and mouse near together to avoid reaching. Your wrists should be straight, with your hands at or slightly below elbow level.

Support: Use a wrist rest if necessary, to keep your wrists in a neutral position.

Accessories:

If your feet cannot comfortably reach the floor, use a footrest.

Document Holder: To avoid neck strain, place documents at eye level next to the monitor.

Posture Tips for Daily Activities

Good posture habits go beyond the workplace. Incorporating these suggestions into your everyday routine can help you stay aligned and avoid discomfort.

Sitting:

Straight Back: Sit with your back straight and your shoulders back. Your buttocks should be touching the back of your chair.

Feet Flat: Place your feet flat on the ground or on a footrest.

Knee Angle: Your knees should be at a straight angle and not crossed.

Standing:

Even Weight Distribution: Stand with your weight evenly distributed over both feet.

Soft Knees: Keep your knees gently bent and not locked.

Your ears, shoulders, and hips should be aligned.

Walking:

Head Up: Keep your head up and your eyes forward.

Keep your shoulders back and relaxed.

Take steady strides and allow your arms to swing naturally.

Lifting:

Proper Technique: Bend at the hips and knees, not your back. Keep the thing close to your body and lift it with your legs rather than your back.

Avoid Twisting: When lifting, turn with your feet rather than twisting your back.

Active Lifestyle Tips

Maintaining an active lifestyle is important for general health and can assist to mitigate the detrimental effects of extended sitting or standing.

Regular Exercise:

Incorporate Variety: Include cardiovascular, strength, and flexibility activities in your workout program.

Aim for at least 150 minutes of moderate-intensity aerobic activity each week, with muscle-strengthening activities on two or more days.

Stretching:

Daily Routine: Stretching should be part of your everyday practice to keep your muscles relaxed and flexible.

Stretch the neck, shoulders, back, hips, and legs.

Integrating Movement Throughout the Day

Breaking up periods of inactivity with movement is critical for overall health and avoiding discomfort.

Take breaks:

Take brief pauses every 30 minutes to stand, stretch, or walk around.

Microbreaks: Take little stretches or walk in place for a minute or two.

Set reminders.

clocks: Use clocks or apps to remind yourself to take regular breaks and walk about.

Standing Desks: Use a standing desk or a desk converter to switch between sitting and standing during the day.

Active Sitting:

Use an exercise ball or a wobbling cushion to strengthen your core muscles while sitting.

Seated activities, such as leg lifts, seated marches, or shoulder rolls, can help you keep physically active.

Balancing Sitting and Standing

Balancing sitting and standing might help your body relax and feel more comfortable.

Alternate positions:

Standing and sitting: Every 30-60 minutes, alternate between the two positions.

Transition Gradually: If you're new to standing desks, start by gradually increasing your standing time to let your body to adjust.

Ergonomic adjustments:

workstation Height: Make sure your workstation is at the appropriate height for both sitting and standing.

Anti-Fatigue Mat: Use an anti-fatigue mat to relieve pressure on your feet and legs while standing.

Posture Awareness:

Check your posture on a regular basis to guarantee optimal alignment, whether you're sitting or standing.

Use Support: When sitting, use back and foot support; when standing, activate your core muscles.

Integrating ergonomic principles and excellent posture habits into your everyday routine can greatly improve your comfort, productivity, and general health. Setting up an ergonomic workspace, maintaining excellent posture, staying active, and balancing sitting and standing can help you avoid discomfort and enhance long-term well-being.

CHAPTER SEVEN

Long-Term Prevention Strategies

To ensure optimal flexibility, strength, and joint health, it is essential to engage in consistent physical activity, follow a balanced diet, and adopt healthy lifestyle practices. By implementing long-term prevention strategies, you can steer clear of injuries, minimize discomfort, and foster a healthier lifestyle.

➤ **Prioritizing Flexibility and Strength**

Consistent Stretching:

Daily routine: Make sure to include stretching in your daily routine to keep your flexibility intact and avoid any muscle tightness.

Areas of Focus: It is important to give careful consideration to stretching the major muscle groups, such as the neck, shoulders, back, hips, and legs.

Strength Training:

Well-rounded Program: Participate in a well-rounded strength training program that focuses on all major muscle groups at least twice a week.

Diverse Range of Exercises: Incorporate a diverse range of exercises to target various muscle groups and minimize the risk of overuse injuries.

Functional Movements:

Include functional exercises that mimic everyday movements to enhance overall strength and coordination.

Some great functional exercises include squats, lunges, push-ups, and planks.

Benefits of Aerobic Exercise:

Weekly Objectives: Strive to achieve a minimum of 150 minutes of aerobic activity per week, either through moderate-intensity exercises like brisk walking or cycling, or through 75 minutes of vigorous-intensity activities like running or aerobics.

Diversify: Incorporate a range of aerobic exercises to maintain a captivating and comprehensive routine.

Strength Training:

Frequency: It is recommended to incorporate strength training exercises into your routine at least two days per week.

Examining Sets and Repetitions: Strive to complete 2-3 sets of 8-12 repetitions for every exercise.

Considering flexibility and balance:

Consider including Yoga and Pilates: Engaging in practices such as yoga and Pilates can enhance flexibility, balance, and core strength.

Balance Exercises: Incorporate balance exercises like standing on one leg or utilizing a balance board.

Developing a strong awareness of your posture is crucial for maintaining a healthy lifestyle.

Pay close attention to your posture throughout the day, whether you're sitting, standing, or walking.

Optimize Your Workspace: Enhance your workspace and daily activities to promote proper posture through ergonomic adjustments.

Breaks for Activities:

Regular Movement: It is important to take regular breaks to move and stretch if you spend long periods sitting.

Consider incorporating a standing desk or an active workstation setup into your routine.

Sleep and Rest:

Make sure to get 7-9 hours of quality sleep each night to give your body the chance to recover and repair.

Include rest days in your exercise routine to avoid overtraining and injuries.

Optimal Nutrition for Joint and Muscle Health

Maintaining a Well-Balanced Diet:

Optimize your diet by incorporating a variety of nutrient-rich foods such as fruits, vegetables, whole grains, lean proteins, and healthy fats.

Consider incorporating anti-inflammatory foods like berries, fatty fish, nuts, and leafy greens into your diet.

Protein Consumption:

Optimal Protein: Make sure your protein intake is sufficient to promote muscle repair and growth. It is important to incorporate a diverse range of protein sources into your diet, such as beans, legumes, tofu, tempeh, nuts, seeds, and plant-based protein powders.

Important Nutrients:

Calcium and Vitamin D are essential for maintaining strong and healthy bones. It is important to make sure you are getting enough of these nutrients in your diet. Make sure to incorporate fortified plant-based milk, leafy greens, and get plenty of sunlight exposure.

Include omega-3 fatty acids in your diet to promote joint health. Sources such as flaxseeds, chia seeds, walnuts, and algae oil supplements are rich in these beneficial nutrients.

Daily Water Consumption:

It is advisable to consume a minimum of 8 cups (64 ounces) of water daily, and even more if you engage in physical activity or reside in hot climates.

Stay on top of your hydration game by always having a water bottle by your side. Don't forget to set reminders to ensure you're getting enough water throughout the day. Boost your hydration levels even further by incorporating water-rich foods like fruits and vegetables into your diet.

Indicators of Dehydration:

Stay vigilant for any indications of dehydration, including urine that is darker than usual, a parched mouth, weariness, and lightheadedness.

It is important to begin hydrating early in the day and maintain consistent hydration levels throughout.

Hydration and Exercise:

Prior to, during, and following exercise, it is crucial to consume water in order to maintain proper hydration levels.

For intense or prolonged exercise sessions, it may be beneficial to consider electrolyte drinks to replenish lost minerals.

Implementing long-term prevention strategies to maintain flexibility and strength requires consistent exercise, a balanced diet, and adopting healthy habits. By implementing these practices into your daily routine, you can enhance your joint and muscle health, minimize the likelihood of injuries, and foster overall well-being. Maintain an active lifestyle, consume a well-rounded diet, stay hydrated, and give importance to your posture and sleep in order to attain a healthier and more active way of living.

END

www.ingramcontent.com/pod-product-compliance
Lightning Source LLC
Chambersburg PA
CBHW071041250726
48653CB00005B/1938